# THE DEATH CARD

# THE DEATH CARD

A Human

Library of Congress Control Number:       2024900385
ISBN:            Softcover              979-8-3694-1443-9
                 eBook                  979-8-3694-1442-2



Print information available on the last page.

Rev. date: 01/11/2024

**To order additional copies of this book, contact:**
Xlibris
844-714-8691
www.Xlibris.com
Orders@Xlibris.com
857846

# CONTENTS

# Part 1

And whenever I look to the future and see myself as an elderly person who maybe suffering from Alzheimer's, looking lost, all around, like someone lost in this world, someone old, incapable and alone…

I say to myself: hey old person, you with your age and poor health with all your difficulties, what do you want from this world and what do you want from this life? What is it that is forcing you to be attached to this life? And what is it about this world that will not leave you alone? From you, an old and lonely person, what is it that it demands? Why is it that it is not leaving you alone to die as you wish?

Why is it that us humans cannot choose for ourselves for how long to endure the old age and the loneliness, and to be able to die when we feel it is time to go? Is this too much to ask for? Can we as an elderly human being choose for ourselves when it is the right time to end our life?

Or is it that there is no end to any journey? Is retirement not an end to the working life? Or night an end to the day? Is not sleep the end to the long and tiresome wakefulness? Is it a problem for us humans to lawfully consider to end our life at a certain age? For example after the age of 80 and after a long life in this world, is it not the right time for an end? A time when we feel it is necessary due to the old age after dealing with ailments, with our own choice?

These thoughts have occupied my mind for years and I have been searching for ways that maybe for myself, and for those who think like me, I could find a way, an answer. A solution so that we do not have to worry about the old age and to live our lives with security and peace of mind. Sometimes the fear of the old age, being incapable and without money, being alone, with Alzheimer's or thousands of other incurable illnesses, shake me so uncontrollably that even the fear of floods, earthquakes, hurricanes and wars would not.

Because age will come for all of us, women and men, black or white, poor and wealthy; and when it comes, it is too late to think about options, unless we have prepared for it in advance.

I do not want to sit and wait around for the old age to come. I do not want to be like the animals who cannot think and without being aware of it, age and die. I want to choose and decide at what age and how to die. Is that not the difference between humans and other creatures, the possibility to think and choose? Perhaps many think about this and tell themselves, why should I worry about the old age in my youth? When I get old, I will die like everyone else; why be concerned with it now when I have my life to live. But I promise you that when they become aware of the details of my ideas, they would volunteer to be first in line.

So I ask you, are you ready for when you are old and incapable or after you have had Alzheimer's, brain aneurysm, or are paralyzed, to have others take care of you? Are you ready to have your children spend their time and life and suffer while tending to you? Are you ready to have your small grandchildren observe your suffering and the suffering of their parents while they care for you? And all of this is only if you have been married and have had children. Have you thought of what would happen if you have not been married and if you have not had children, and if you have not saved enough money to take care of your expenses during your old age? Are you hopeful that social services and the help of the government would be the solution to these problems?

Is it not time that as human beings we think about our old age, loneliness, the incapability of our bodies and our minds and to find a simpler solution that would not only benefit us, but would also benefit those around us, our world and the society?

"Part between part 1 and part 2"

Sometimes I think to myself if I want to die in my old age, do I have to ask for someone's permission or get a license to die? If so, why?

Why can I not be able to choose that when I am old and alone, or if I am above 80 years old to choose to stay or not, to live or die? Is it an impossible wish to choose to end my life legally? is there a timeline, a time at which point, for example when 80 years old, that us humans can choose for ourselves to end our life if we want? And would the law help me, and those who think like me, once an old age is reached to choose a calm and peaceful end to our pain and suffering?

# Part 2

I remember a time when I had a long conversation with a friend, talking about the subject, I asked how would you like to die when you get old?

With a smile she replied, of course it's clear. I would like to have a peaceful death, with no pain, and without being sick for a long time, without suffering. As they used to say, I would like to go to sleep one night and to not wake up the next day.

I said many people like this type of dying when they are old and incapable, then why can we not create a process where we can have this kind of death?

My friend replied, the way you talk, you think it is that simple?

I said it might be simpler than you think, maybe before nobody thought about it or if they have, it was in a way that was not acceptable by others.

My friend replied and now you think you have found a way?

I said I think so... I have some ideas but I want to see if they work before I get old and others become in charge of how I can die. My friend seemed curious so I continued, the same way that we have identity cards to be able to give blood or to give our body parts after our death, I have been thinking about a card, "the death card." It would be a card that by signing up for it, when at an advanced age, maybe above 80, or when one is diagnosed with Alzheimer's, paralyzed or diagnosed with an incurable illness, or even if you are old and alone and do not want to continue living, you would have the right to choose to die legally. It would be that simple.

My friend said I am a bit confused but even if I accept what you are saying, do you think it would be that simple?

I replied, when a new idea has come about, at first, many are against it.

It takes a while for people to get used to it, similar to the way that giving your blood to save someone else's life came about. At first, many were against it. Or when the physicians wanted people to understand that they could donate their body parts after their death, and by donating a part of themselves they could save someone from death, many were vehemently against it. It took a long time and still many are not accepting and do not volunteer their own body parts after their death. But my point is that the law has given us the chance to choose to give our blood and our body parts; it is completely legal.

So I want to try and see if we can earn the right to choose at old age, maybe above 80, even if we are healthy but we do not want to live any longer, that we can choose for ourselves. Is it not fair that when an elderly person wants to live, if they want to continue their life by any unnatural means, they have the right to do so? Why should it not be the other way around?

My friend said then you think in the future, people can choose their time of death and the method of their death legally? Even if that older person is healthy and for whatever reason decides not to continue living?

I replied it would become so common that people would forget that before it was a different way. Then without being able to stop myself from laughing I said, even after I am 80 and have a healthy mind and am active, I would like to donate my brain so they could use it for another person.

My friend laughed and said now you have gone too far, plus who would want your brain?

I said you can laugh at me, but I am quite serious. There will be a time when brain transplants can be done and why not use my brain? Imagine if a young person is dying from brain injury, but the rest of their body is healthy and there is only the need for a healthy brain. Why not use the brain of an 80 year old, if it is healthy?

Although I am not sure who would benefit from that. The younger person or the older one or even if it would be possible. Then laughing I continued, if it were possible, the older persons brain would have a new body and the younger person, without any trials, could benefit from the experiences of the elder person's brain. I wonder if the old brain, after seeing that it now possesses a new body, would become young again or is it that the younger body would force it's rights on the older person's brain? Does anyone know?

"Part between part 2 and part 3"

It appears that every one hundred years something new occurs in our world that we have no choice but to accept it. It is because the time for the idea has come. But maybe similar to the chicken and the egg dilemma, it is complicated; not knowing which came first. Is it that a new idea emerges and then people accept the new idea, or is it that the circumstances change to necessitate that a new idea emerge to solve the issue at hand and then it comes about.

# PART 3

Someone may ask me, are you capable of leaving your grandfather, grandmother or your parents who are inflicted by an illness, paralyzed or have Alzheimer's in an institution where they would end their lives? Are you so cruel?

My answer to the question is that I would never make that decision for them or anyone else. I am not responsible for other peoples lives. It is important and I have to repeat that I only want to make this decision for myself. It has been these types of wrong assumptions that has been the stumbling block for ideas such as this. Because one way or another others think they would have to make the decision for the other people and they are worried about confronting resistance from others, and even getting cursed by the members of the society and those close to them. This is an idea that I have for my own future and I would like to set the groundwork so that for me, and those who think alike, this would be a possibility.

I am only voicing my own idea and depending on others views, they can choose for themselves on how they would want to die. And it is with sadness that I have to say, that if I start an institution that could carry out what I am hoping to set up, it would only be for me and the young people who would want to make this decision for when they reach an older age, who could join and get the "the death card". This would mean that the elderly, incapable and incapacitated people would not be able to use the services of this institution. It would be hard to see the elderly who would be looking with envy at the peacefulness that we experience, but that cannot be helped. Maybe they would say to themselves, why is it that no one sat up this institution at the time of our youth, so that we could benefit from the benefits of such arrangements and not suffer from pain and endure the waiting of an uncertain future.

No one knows why people wait for until the pain and suffering begins and then think of what needs to be done. And why when people see someone is working to find a solution to help themselves and others, they would create obstacles to stop them? Is the fear from becoming old, finding the route to progress, and finding peace not important that no one could think of a solution?

## "Part between part 3 and part 4"

I have always been fascinated by the life of the animals and always think what a comfortable life they have, living day by day, sleeping, raising their young and then death, without knowing or being capable of changing anything or having any concerns about their future. They are only concerned about the present, they do not look back to the past or to the future.

However as humans, with our reasonings and the power of our thoughts, we cannot wait around for events to take place naturally, without us trying to affect the outcome.

We can see the past and the elderly who have lived with pain, suffering and loneliness before passing on. We can project into the future and see how we could be one of those people incapable and alone and we cannot sit around for the old age to arrive and like being stuck in the marsh or quicksand slowly drown.

We have the depth of our knowledge, we can choose and create change, we can separate ourselves from the other creatures and take control of our own lives and our own futures.

# Part 4

I was thinking about the subject, contemplating what I would call this institution. I want this institution to have a name that would feel good to me and to those who would be interested in participating in it. Maybe a name such as the "last station", the "last visit", or the "last house" would be good. But no, the word "last" does not bring about good feelings. It has the connotation of sadness or saying good bye. So maybe the "death celebration", the "song of death", or the "dance of death". No, maybe death at an old age and incapability philosophically seem right, but it accompanies sadness and I do not believe any of these names portray a good picture. No, I do not believe any name that has a negative feeling associated with this concept would work.

When someone wants to go on a trip, before taking the trip, they make arrangements. There is excitement and happy feelings with the planning, so maybe the word "travel" could be used.

"Trip to eternity", "trip to new worlds" have better feelings to them. For now, I would call this institution "trip to eternity". Now that I have chosen a name, I need to see if I can attract investors. Can I get the help of the federal government? At first, I have to see what would be important for a country to be interested in this concept, obviously governments are interested in returns on any investments.

First I have to see what ideas are important to a governmental institution. What is certain is that ideas that produce income are of interest to them. So, I would need to raise their interest by considering a profitable venture. With that in mind, I thought about what kind of money a government can make, if we elderly want to voluntarily die at a certain age? When the government becomes aware that many of when elderly would voluntarily get "the death card" so that when we want to end our lives, would they then become interested. Why? Well, the income from those who plan their death would be gone, and so would all their expenses.

Secondly, there will not be as much need for elderly facilities, hospital care, hospice and all the other associated organizations. So would the cost of the doctors, nurses and medicines be gone. Then the governments can spend all that money on all the other needs of their societies. So eliminate the cost of the elderly care and allocate the funds for other needs.

Maybe the funds could be used to help the teenagers who are often forgotten, those who need assistance for education, recreational activities, academic and artistic endeavors, where there is so much need. I am certain that not I, nor those who think like me, would choose spending funds on lengthening their lives at an old age versus caring for the teenagers. So should a younger person like me, who chooses to let go and die, stay at the cost of the others? And what of the young who are in need, without any hope or help and commit suicides? Did we not humans set the rules of law to govern the society and the health of our societies?

## "Part between part 4 and part 5"

I see many teenagers and young adults spending their youth entertaining themselves by partying, drinking, using drugs and the assortments of the "feel good" pills. Many lose their lives from these activities and the use of these substances. So who is responsible for the loss of these assets in our society? Why is it that mostly the children of the wealthy are able to benefit from good education, artistic and physical education and activities? Is it not time for the governments to stop wasting money to enforce the care for the elderly, for people like me and those who think like me, who prefer to end our lives when they get old?

The funds spent for the care of the elderly who do not want to continue living could be used to fund the care for our teenagers, the way I, and those like minded individuals, believe. Why are there limited resources to advise, care and educate those teenagers who are the assets of our societies?

If people support their governments, then the governments should support the wishes of their citizens. The government cannot leave all of the responsibilities of raising the teenagers to their parents. Parents who do their best to provide for their children and work and work and work, and as a result, seldom have the capability to tend to all the aspects of their children's well-being. The government and the parents need to work together to protect and prepare their teens to build better societies.

# Part 5

Some may think that if someone wants to voluntarily die at an old age, is that not really a form of suicide? In answer I would say, maybe it would seem that way but in reality to save a society and for the peace of mind of the person, it may be necessary for people and the society to accept the wishes of another even if that seems unusual to them.

Is this not similar to when there is a war between two countries, the soldiers fight fiercely and some sacrifice their lives to save the lives of their comrades? Is that not a form of suicide? For those who work in dangerous caves or the people who handle radioactive materials, is that not a form of suicide? there are many forms of activities such as flying, driving on the freeways at a high speed, and some times under the influence of alcohol or drugs, others while eating excessive unhealthy sweets and fatty foods and even breathing the unhealthy and dangerous air in the busy metropolitan cities. Are not all of these forms of suicide?

If we are honest with ourselves we will see that one way or another we are committing a form of suicide, whether we know or not...! Sometimes it may seem a slow and quiet process and we may not even be aware of it happening. And even if we die slowly and quietly, is that not a form of suicide? Having an accident, is that not a form of suicide? But no accidents are quick and we are not aware of it until they happen. So when we are dying and we are not aware of it, it is not suicide, but if we and others know it, then it is suicide?

Looking at it in this manner, does anyone really die from natural death anymore? It is because we have turned everything from natural to unnatural these days. We no longer live in a jungle, sleeping, eating, reproducing or dying in a natural habitat. So in that sense, living in an unnatural world, would it make sense to think of dying in a natural way? Would it not be fair for me to have the permission to die unnaturally in an unnatural world, even if some people call that suicide?

## "Part between part 5 and part 6"

I do not remember where I read or heard that scientists were trying to kill cancerous tumors by turning them to become suicidal, in order to not harm the healthy cells around them.

So even if in theory, it is interesting to me that if I decide at an old age to become a cancerous tumor and turn onto myself, in order to help myself and those around me, it would be called suicide.

# Part 6

Yesterday we were gathered at a company auditorium listening to an insurance representative who was explaining the benefits of having insurance. Some in the audience were skeptical of what they were hearing.

The beautiful mixed race lady who was making the presentation had a big smile on her face all throughout her presentation, showing off her more than natural white teeth as she spoke. Her teeth seemed fake and it was unusual the way she was showing them off as she spoke. Typically when someone speaks, their face show a mix of emotions. She even smiled widely as she spoke about sickness, hospital stay, accident, death and the enormous costs of recovery. I did not understand what she was smiling about most of the time.

She spoke about the different types of insurance, insurance for the individual, their spouse and family and how the cost of insurance was going up and up constantly. She spoke about how by paying a higher premium, we could enjoy the services of better doctors, ambulance, accident recovery, surgery and hospital. I thought to myself the cost of covering for insurance is going to soon be higher than our salaries. While looking around, I saw the worried faces of most of my colleagues and their discomfort in what they were hearing. There were different age people in the audience and the more older individuals, the more worried they seemed. Because as it was being presented, the cost of covering a younger person was not as high as the insurance premium for an older individual. She kept continuing to talk with her big smile on her face.

I was getting bored and began wondering. I thought to myself, with the costs as high as they are, it is better we do not get sick, better not do much in order to prevent from getting injured. It seemed the only option was to just go ahead and lie down and die. I thought to myself if I start my Institute of "trip to eternity", what kind of a person I would send around to provide information and advertise the concepts of the institution? Would people then listen with interest or with worry? Would they not be happy to know that by joining this institution, they would not have to worry about all the expenses that an old person would have to plan for? Would they be happy to know that after working for most of their lives, they would not have to cover the costs of the medical services, hospital, nurses and expensive medications? Would they be happy to know that they can leave something behind for their children when it was time? Would it not be of value that when we are young and have "the death card", paying a small fee to the "trip to eternity" institution, we would not have to worry about our old age? Would that not be a pleasurable thought?

When I came out of my own pondering, I looked around and everyone was still listening to the presentation without any smiles on their faces. If someone looked, they would see a smile on my face, perhaps, but it was a sad smile for myself and my colleagues who could not see a way out except to accept the high cost of the insurance. I felt like I was in a marsh, sinking deep without being able to move. All I could do was to hang on to any nearby branch to try to stay where I was and to not drown completely.

Maybe when illness and all the suffering occurs for ourselves, or for those dear to us, it would not matter what the costs are and whether or not insurance covers the needed care. We would spend all our savings to cover what needs to be taken care of. Of course I do not deny the need for insurance, because it gives us the peace of mind, but it is hard to understand why they have to cost so much. It seems as though there is no sense of humanity, except spending and spending and spending, when it comes to insurance. Maybe when I start the "trip to eternity" institute, I would need to think about not having hefty cost associated with it and to make sure it would be affordable. Of course if I have any say so in the matter. Maybe I would need to try to make this be a governmental institution, rather than a private institution, would I have any power in determining that? I really do not know.

"Part between part 6 and part 7"

So we may have another monthly cost in the future for the "death card" for our old age. I am certain that the same concerns about death at an old age, similar to what it is now, would still be present. I would think at that time, there would be fewer people thinking and worrying about all these matters, because they have planned for it in advance.

# PART 7

When I am at a gathering and the time is right, I try to expertly turn the conversation to the issues about old age, issues such as loneliness, incurable illnesses and so on. As the conversation progresses, I present my idea about the "death card" and the "trip to eternity" institute and having a choice in how and when we die. I am interested in hearing the pros and cons from different people about this idea.

At one of these gatherings, someone asked me would the person who would perform the final act of the injecting the powerful and deadly dose not be called a murderer?

I answered, looking comfortably at him, it depends from what point of view you are looking at it.

He asked what do you mean?

I said, when justice declares the death penalty to an individual, would the person who would be carrying out the final ruling be considered a murderer? At the time of war, when a soldier kills an opposing enemy soldier, is that soldier a murderer? In both of these scenarios, the person who gets killed did not want to die. Compare that to a scenario when by having a "death card" and choosing that route when I am completely capable of making decisions for myself, and choose to die at an age of 80, or later. So if someone does their job with love, while preserving my rights, would that person then be considered a murderer? When you think about it in that manner, this would be a job, like any other job. When someone dutifully performs their role, it is just like any other job. We would not then call that person a murderer. Then jokingly I added, of course if everything goes as planned and I get the rights to the "trip to eternity" institution, when someone has a problem with this issue, maybe we can use a robot to give the final injection. As we know robots would not have any problem carrying out what needs to be done.

My belief is that when the time comes and people feel comfortable with this concept, everything would go quickly and people would forget that in a time before this, people would wait around until death came their way. And that in many cases, we would keep an ill old person waiting for a long long time. In the future, the elderly can choose the time of their own death and end this dictatorship governance of death.

## "Part between part 7 and part 8"

It has only been a few weeks since I started writing this book, and I have started to have some negative thoughts that have prevented me from continuing my writing. There is a voice in my head asking, why are you trying to disrupt the order to the natural world? Why are you fighting with death? Why do you want to control death?

Why do you not want to allow death to come as it pleases and take people at an old age at any time it wants? Why do you want to be the one who chooses how and when to die after the age of 80? And why are you trying to encourage others to make this decision as well? There are many questions that are occupying my mind, some even making fun of me. It seems like there is a power that comes from somewhere barring me from continuing on my quest. But this time I have made a decision and I have began a journey into this realm, and until I reach a point that satisfies me, I cannot stop. Even if I can only carry out this idea for myself legally. Maybe it seems selfish to not want to take others along with me, but do I have the right to encourage others to decide to die at a planned old age? Even if this decision is a legal one and makes living our lives happier by being in control, without thinking, worrying and the fear of loneliness and death at an old age?

# Part 8

I remember the day I was at the gas station and waiting my turn I saw that the car in front of me belonged to an elderly couple. I was watching them calmly and the way the older lady was showing the older man how to use his card to get gas. Why, I do not know. It did not seem like an important event, but as I was watching them I could not help notice the trembling hands of the older man and how he had trouble pulling the card out quickly as it was required. Over and over, again and again he tried and he was getting the error message. The car in front of them drove away and the driver behind me asked, are you going forward? I gestured by hand, to let him know that he could go forward in front of them.

I watched as the older gentleman tried over and over to enter the code and to pull out the card on time, without any success. I wonder if the people who design these cards think about the elderly who have to be able to work with these machines with their trembling hands. I am not sure why the older gentleman was trying to do this by himself and why he was not getting any help from the attendant.

As I watched them, I thought to myself would I reach that age when I need help to continue with my daily activities? A car horn brought me to myself as another driver behind me was asking if I wanted to go ahead of the elderly couple as the place in front of them was vacant again. Again, I gestured that if you wanted to, he could go forward. Finally, the gas station attendant who had become aware of what was going on came forward and politely asked if he could help pump gas for the couple. I thought to myself, now they will be going home maybe after running their errands on their way; then tired, they would prepare something to eat along with taking a lot of pills and medicines. Maybe they would turn on the tv and watch something and talk to each other, repeating their repetitive memories and stories of their past to one another. Maybe they would hear from a child or a friend, and after resting their old and tired feet, hands and backs, they would wait for the night time to arrive, so they could eat their dinner, take their medications and go to sleep. Only to wake up the next day with the same pains and aches and start a new day just like the previous one. They will repeat this process over and over until death comes their way and takes them away from this tiresome lives. And this is the life of the elderly who are capable of moving about and are somewhat in good health, not those who have Alzheimer's, and paralyzed and cannot move around, without children, friends or money. Again the honk of a car horn behind me brought me back, and I was thinking of gesturing again for the car to go ahead of me, when I realized the older couple had left, so I moved forward to get gas.

———

## "Part between part 8 and part 9 (a)"

Sometimes I think I take life too seriously and I should bring a sense of humor to my thoughts. So I thought, how would someone choose when it would be a good season, day of the week, or time of day or night to die? I think I would prefer to die in the spring, when it is neither warm nor cold, rather than choosing to die in the cold and snowy weather or in a hot summer day. This way the people who would come to my funeral would be comfortable.

I would not want to die in the beginning of the week, because that is when people start their own week. End of the week would not be a good time either, because that is the time when people go out and would want to relax and enjoy their weekend. So I think the middle of the week would be a good time for dying. People would tell each other, did you hear... so and so is dead...

But maybe some people would prefer to go to a funeral at the end of the week so that they would not have to take a day off in order to attend the funeral ceremony. So maybe it would be good in order to cause trouble, to die in the middle of the week, on a snowy and very cold day, just to see who actually cared about me. And about the time of the death, morning, noon, or night? I do not believe in dying in the morning after waking up from a long and deep sleep, would not be when I would want to take my final journey to eternity. How about noon? Maybe after eating a really delicious lunch, it would not be bad to take a nice long nap. I have heard from many, that when they get old, they would want to go to sleep at night and to not wake up the next day. So maybe it would be good when we reach the old age, one night at the end of the week, on a nice summer day, that would be when I would close my eyes and go to sleep and not wake up the next day.

## "Part between part 8 and part 9 (b)"

Maybe it is time for me to talk about the parts between the various parts of my book. To tell the truth, after writing a chapter, several days go by and without having started the next chapter, ideas come to my mind that relate to what I have already written. I do not like to go back and change what I have already written. I do not want to change my mind about what I have written and to take out or add parts to what I have already written. So I decided on having the parts in between, so that I can continue my thoughts about what I have already written in the previous chapter.

## "Part between part 8 and part 9 (c)"

I can only write at the time I have for lunch when I am at work, that is when I can concentrate sitting in my car and writing what is on my mind. Sometimes I finish a part, or sometimes I can only write a part of it and I need to continue it on another day or the next. If I were to compare my process to the work of a painter, I would say that it is like a painter who would work on a painting on two or three different days at a specific time allocated for that work to finish. Or it can be compared to a painter who works on three different paintings, such as it is fashionable now, where they would be placed on the wall next to one another. In order to complete the work and since on different days the light and the weather has changed, there may be differences between these three pieces of work that will keep them somewhat apart.

So will my writings be the same? Does that mean that my writings may appear to be connected, but in reality they are not?

# Part 9

A few days ago I was walking by the lake near my house, looking around at the lake, the ducks swimming around in the water, the mountains surrounding the area far away. I was watching the people walking around the lake alone or with others when I saw an old man pushing his spouse's wheel chair. They stopped by the lake in front of me and I slowed my steps and came near them as I watch the lake and smiled. The old man smiled back, but there were no changes in the old woman's face. Some of the ducks came by our way, thinking we were going to feed them. I went over to the ducks and jokingly said, what is it that you want, food? The ducks realizing I had nothing to give them began swimming away. The old man had a friendly smile on his face. I looked at the old woman and saw that her face had no recognition of anything, just a blank stare. I felt like she was not really seeing the lake, nor the ducks or anyone else. She seemed like a plant that seemed to need sunlight, fresh air and some water and nothing else.

I said it is a beautiful day. He agreed by shaking his head up and down and said, I have brought my wife out to get some fresh air, although…

I asked how long has she been sick? He said it has been a year since she had brain aneurysm and has become paralyzed, since then she is neither better nor worse. Sometimes when I look at her I do not recognize her, there is no more life in her eyes.

I said, I understand it is difficult, my grandfather suffered from a similar condition. I asked do you have any children to help you and to visit?

He said we have one child who lives far away in another city with his own family, we do not have much expectations.

I asked so you are the only caretaker for your wife?

He said, no there is a nurse who comes daily to help with our daily needs and leaves.

I asked, do you have friends who can visit with you?

With a sad smile, he said most of them are in similar situations and are dealing with their own illnesses, pains or loneliness. Some are living in senior care and others in hospitals and yet others are dead. He stopped talking and showed much pain in his face, so respecting his quiet, I continued looking at the lake.

After a while I asked him some couples think that when they are old, like above the age of 80, they would want to leave this world together. What do you think?

He said many think that after years of living together with love, when they are old and incapable, that it would be better for them to die together and to not leave each other alone. It would be difficult to live alone after having had someone in your life for so long. Of course that is a dream for many.

I said, I believe as impossible as it may seem, that there would be a future where it would be legal for us to have such a choice.

He smiled and said it may be a dream, but it may be too late for my wife and I and, and out of our reach. But I would be happy to know that others would not suffer from pain, loneliness and enduring what comes with the old age.

I looked at his wife and saw that while we had been talking, there was nothing, no reaction from her, except for the infinite quiet. I was thinking to myself, looking at the quiet of the lake, when I came to myself and realized that they were gone. I did not remember if I said goodbye or not. Sometimes I go deep into my thoughts and forget the outside world and do not even hear any sounds around me.

## "Part between part 9 and part 10 (a)"

It has been years since this idea has come to my mind, sometimes I would forget about it for a long time, but it would come back and occupy my mind, forcing me to continue thinking about it. I could not decide if I should introduce my idea to anyone or not or whether or not to ask for anyone's help? The first time I thought about this idea, I wrote a short story, which I shared with my publisher who discouraged me from publishing my story. I do not know why…. but after a few years of not thinking about it, the idea came back to me again and it no longer wanted to stay hidden in a far corner of my mind.

It seemed like it wanted to tell me it is not so simple for you to think of an idea that would make the world a better place, to then not do anything about it and to move on with your life and die. It seemed as if it was saying that when idea comes to someone and remain dormant that anyone can then pick up the idea and begin working on it. So now that you have been haunted by it and have spent years thinking about it for so many years, it is time to continue working on it. You have made this idea come alive in your mind and cannot allow it to die. You must do something and you do not have the right to give it up. It is time to move on. That is why I decided to sit down and begin doing something about it.

So I thought to myself it is time and what are some of the ways I could go about it? I could have first registered my idea and looked for some investors. But how when I did not have any experience in that field. Then I thought of writing a script and proposing my idea to someone for making a movie, but I was not a script writer. Maybe I could go and begin talking about it in front of others, more than just talking to friends, but I really did not have any background in public speaking. So what remained was what I could do and that was writing a book. Some say that books have lost their power and they are fewer and fewer people reading these days, but I could not lose hope.

When I thought about writing, I thought of many who write books in order to showcase their ideas and their beliefs, so even though I was not hopeful I decided to begin writing. But what kind of a book could I write? A short story, a long story, a novel or series of books? Would it be better for the main character in my book to be an old man who was suffering from Alzheimer's, was paralyzed or had gone crazy? Or an old person who was over 80 years old, enduring aches and pains and lives alone? How would others react to such stories, except by shedding some tears at the end of the story? Shedding a few tears when millions are alone and old? Old age and issues relating to it will come my way and yours, and if we are late taking any action, we would be that same old and lonely person. I remembered a long time ago when I had a sad problem, crying did not solve my problem. I thought to myself then, that if my problem would get solved by crying, I would gladly cry for days, but I knew better. And for that reason I did not want to write a book that would make others cry, without coming up with some solutions to the issues. I wanted to take a different approach and instead of making a sad film portraying the life of an old person who was suffering from illness and living a lonely life, to write a book that could propose some solutions.

I thought maybe it would not be a bad idea to start my story in the future, maybe 500 years from now and to show a world where people have the "death card", similar to having a card for donating blood, identifying a blood donor or a card for donating body parts. That way when they are old, incapable and lonely, when they are ready to die, they can legally contact the institute and legally end their lives. At that time this would be a common event that no one would even think twice about. Of course there are always people who do not like this idea and they would want to live and die naturally, but I doubt there would be many. This would still be similar to donating blood, such as it was common in the past where people would die from simple injuries because of the loss of blood. It is also similar to when people did not think of donating their body parts even if brain dead to save the lives of others who needed a body part to continue their lives, which is miraculous. And even to this day there are others who would not donate their own blood or body parts, but not many. Of course it is a personal choice for people to do as they please with their blood and body parts. So I decided in writing a book to present my idea would be a good start.

So what type of book would I write? I thought of years ago, when my first book, which was a collection of my short stories was published. I remembered someone read a story and began criticizing what I had written and began attacking my character and my beliefs. This was done by my own colleagues at a book club where they knew me, by people who had not yet published any of their own work but they believed that they were better than me. This had such a negative effect on me that for a long time I did not write anything more. But the good thing that happened is that before leaving, a respected gentleman approached me and said "this is my phone number if you would like, please contact me. And continued before leaving, "I saw many good things in your writing, I saw the talent and I believe you will write many better books. Please contact me" and left.

I called him a few weeks later when I had calmed down. He said, " as I understand it from your writing style, you know the basics of writing, you know the styles and structure of the story and you have taken courses in storytelling but unfortunately that is creating some confusion in your writing. Your stories are composed of strong parts that originate from the fluidity of your mind, along with weak parts that you seem to have forced into your writing based on what you have learned. That has hurt your whole story and your story does not seem to coherent."

He continued, "when you have an interesting idea, continue writing about it… then maybe leave it aside and go back to it after a while and keep editing until it is ready."

So now after several years, I have began writing and I want to write the way I was told without concern for other people's opinions. I just want to write and to express my ideas and thoughts. Maybe this is not the best way to go, but it is what I can do for now, so I began and I know I have a long way to go and hope that I will succeed.

## "Part between part 9 and 10 (b)"

I believe it is time for me to write my opinion about writers, I have my opinion about writers of story books, not other types of writers....

I would like to explain what I think, in my opinion, if you divide people into two groups "general" and "specific" and I don't mean the inventors, founders or researchers who bring about something new, that than the "general" people go about their daily and pre- programmed lives. And then there is a third group, whom I call the "in between" the two, who neither wish to obey the everyday ways of life in the society, nor wish to be involved in solving any issues. These are the ones who are writers, with their active minds, sometimes find their way in with the "general" and sometimes in the "specific" group. They think more and see what is going on in the society and sometimes suffering from hopelessness and their need to get away from the pain of what they see, commit suicide. Sometimes while at the height of stardom, wealth and comfort they take their own life, because they are the only ones who know their own suffering, they are suffering from what they have hidden from many.

One of the pains of these writers is that they are never happy with their own work, their writing, even though others find them their work amazing. Most writers have two sides to them, one is their outside persona, strong and confident, and the other is their internal persona, which is broken and lacks confidence. They know who they are, they know they think differently than others, writing with excitement, and yet they reach midway or sometimes at the end of their work, feel tired and helpless. Once their work reaches the second or third rounds of publication, they would angrily throw away book and resume their daily lives, trying to just forget the excitement that they felt before. The ones who can come back and start writing again, are the lucky ones.

# PART 10

Where would be a good place to stay, before death, at the old age when we decide to go? I am speaking about a place that after receiving the "death card" from the "trip to eternity" institute, when the time has come that we feel it is the moment that we would want to die. Should it be a place like a hospital or like a rest home?

I would want to spend the last moments and days of my life in a happy and comfortable place, maybe like a hotel. What do you think? It would be a place that you would go for a few days to rest and visit with friends or relatives, if you want to say goodbye. Just like when we are going on a trip, of course we would not be returning from this trip. Because the destination for this trip, where we will all eventually end up, whether it is preplanned or not, and whether we like it or not. So I ask you, would you go on a long trip without making any preparations? Don't most people plan and make preparations before going on a trip? Of course we do, because we are humans and we have the choice to choose where we want to go to, just as we will soon be able to choose the time of our death in our old age.

Of course I am not talking about the sudden or accidental death, because those are events that we cannot plan for, and we cannot prevent from accidental death. But it does not mean that we cannot make preparations for when we actually choose to go. So let us go back to thinking about the building and whom we would want to be working there. Would we be able to use the same doctors and nurses as there are in the hospitals or would we need to choose and train individuals specifically to work in this institution? So would it require that we have new fields of study at the University or maybe a short certificate program at colleges?

I would think we would need psychologist, those who can speak with the individuals who choose this program. But I do not believe that for those who like to go this route, they would change their mind, but we better consider that. There are those who cancel or change their mind at the last minute, even if this trip is the "trip to eternity", so we need to account for that.

And for some who would be there for a few days, there maybe a need for doctors and nurses to take care of them in intensive care. Some may facetiously say that if someone is going to die, why would they need special care?

In answer I would say, if I arrange for everything, it would be so that those who have chosen to go this route, would not want to feel any pain. I would want to be comfortable on their last days of my life. In my mind, the reason for the staff is so that no one would be alone or in pain. I agree with the injection of a strong and calmative medication that would cause drowsiness and then a peaceful death. But I am not sure what type of education this person would need in order to provide this function. I am not talking about the act of actually giving the injection, but for their psychological needs to be able to calmly perform.

I am not aware of the type of education, if any, which is provided for the people who perform many of the jobs such as the hanging, electric chair execution, guillotine or in the firing squad.

The difference here would be that the person who is convicted of a crime does not want to die, whereas in this case the person has decided to voluntarily die at an old age does. In the first case, the person who has committed a crime, whether because of their genetics, environment or what has happened in their lives has behaved in a manner that the society finds them guilty, does not want to die. That person would want to be treated and to continue living, but the society decides that this person deserves to die. But in the second case, the old person who has made preparations for years to die at an age of 80 years or older, would not want to live any longer. That person would just want to be able to legally end their life without the interference of anyone else. Now, it is the others and the society that insistently want that old person to live and to continue living a life full of suffering.

Do you not think that we live in a crazy world? Is it not time to review our old ways of thinking and to change our decrepitated laws? Is it not time to bring humanity for the comfort of our elderly? Sometimes I think to myself, when we humans convict someone to death, are we not sinners? And what of when we force an elderly person to continue living, despite all of their pains and sufferings?

## "Part between part 10 and part 11 (a)"

Sometimes I am surprised by my own ideas and patterns of thoughts, and I wonder why I cannot write about them the way I see them in my mind? I think something impedes and prevents us from transferring our thoughts into words and I wonder if it is self made? This may be one of the biggest fears that may be affecting many writers, by not allowing them to write freely, without any fears and worries about the society, race, gender, religion, work or place.

Unfortunately this almost prevented me from writing about my ideas freely, thinking I should choose a pen name for writing this book, a name like "A human". In that way, no one would wonder about my gender, place of origin, religion, job, or societal status and who I am. Then they would not try to prevent me from writing this book. And even if this book earns an award, the prize would belong to the book itself and not to anyone in particular. Why do people always wonder where the writer is from? Why do they not say the writer is a human from the planet earth? Maybe in the future, this would be the case, when we meet other creatures from other planets.

Also, I am thinking that in writing under the pen name of "a human", I would preserve my privacy and I would not need to deal with the outreach of journalists, and others would not know the details of my life. That way, I can live my own life and come up with my own ideas that would pertain to the every day issues, similar to the experience I had at the book club that I mentioned before. I do not know how other writers like to live after the publication of their book, but I belong to the group that prefers to continue a normal life. I would not want to be forced into seclusion because of the thoughts and opinions of the others. I do not want others and their opinions to affect my writings. Otherwise, I may end up writing a book that would only interest the "specifics", not for the "general ", and not even for myself.

---

## "Part between part 10 and part 11 (b)"

I go to work at a specific time every morning. Sometimes as I am driving to work, I take a road where there is a slight downhill gradient. This street is long and without any turns, so I can see a long way ahead of me. Almost every day I see an old man walking along the road, with his skinny legs that are somewhat bent, carrying a cane and walking with a light brown colored dog. They always attract my attention and as I get close, I slow down to look at their movement as I pass by them. Sometimes I think to myself, which one of these really needs the other? Is it the old man who had brought his dog for the fresh air or is it the dog that has brought the old man for the fresh air? Is it the old man who is following the dog or is it the dog following the old man? I do not know why these thoughts occupy my mind so much and what they want to tell me? Maybe it is feeling the pain, the loneliness and the feelings of the elderly peoples! Every day I think about this and I cannot find an answer, but I wonder, they are the living characters of my book? How long will they survive? I do not know...

# Part 11

Some may ask, why is it that I so enthusiastically seek answers for my idea? Why is it that I cannot continue to live, just like others, and to die when I reach an old age? My answer to these questions is love. Love for myself, love for my future, and love for those who think like me. Those who are waiting for someone to take the first step and in a loud and without any fear would say, "I would like to be able to die legally at an old age, when I am incapable and alone, and when I want to." After that, others will follow.

The same people who always look and wait for someone to find ways and solutions and then follow them. These are the people that slowly, or sometimes quickly, accept everything and without any questions volunteer to be the first. Now I ask you, does not love mean loving ourselves? Love for our physical body and our mind…Can we love others without loving ourselves?

Is it right that we have to live our lives with the fear for our old age? While we can set the ground work and have the peace of mind. In the same manner that we get insurance, whether it be health insurance, disability insurance, life insurance, house or car insurance and so on for the peace of mind, we can also get the "death card" for our old age.

Would we want for our family, over many years to have to care for us and to have to suffer, physically and mentally, while we do not even want to continue living when old?

I remember many years ago, I was at a funeral service of an acquaintance, someone who had suddenly passed from a heart attack. Talking to a respectable and educated lady, who was one of my acquaintances, she said, lucky him, what a great way to go, without any pain or suffering and without causing any suffering for those around him.

I said it really is true, many like to die that way.

She said, this is how I would want to go to, with a heart attack when I get old, or while crossing the street for a speeding truck to take me out and for me to die suddenly.

I looked at her with surprise, because to me that seemed like a terrible way to die...., I wondered why would such an educated and respectable lady like her think to die in that manner? So I asked her and she answered, I have a brother who has been suffering from Alzheimer's for many years. He was a university professor and now does not understand anything and cannot even take care of his own daily care. He needs care from many people, nurses and relatives and he is spending his old age in such a sad way. With a big sigh she continued, I would never want to be like him, to spend my old age in that unbearable way.

So I understood why she would even consider a tragic way of dying. Is it not time we think about our old age and make the preparations so that we can spend our lives calmly and without any fear of the future?

## "Part between part 11 and part 12 (a)"

Sometimes I see someone working hard to acquire properties, constantly investing in all sorts of ways, and I ask what is the reason for all this and the need to make so much money? The answer I get is that we can never have enough because we do not know what will happen when we are old, what expenses we would have, what illnesses we have to deal with. So while we can, we must make as much money as we can and to save as much as possible for our futures.

This is why I wish to plan for my future, so that when I am old, incapable, lonely and reach the age of 80, when I feel that my daily life needs other's help, and that I am not able to do anything more in this world, to be able to legally end my life in the "trip to eternity" Institute. And I think to myself, by choosing to die legally at an old age, I can live and not waste my life, with all the fears of having to deal with the old age expenses. Would I not be a more useful human being in that case?

"Part between part 11 and part 12 (b)"

Maybe one of the advantages of getting "the death card" early on in our lives, would be so that when we get old and if we lose our mental capacity, we can arrange for the "trip to eternity" institute to make the arrangements to end our lives. Our relatives can then carry out our wishes by contacting the institute, without any guilt. That way, there would not be any hard feelings or any doubt for the pre-arranged death.

# Part 12

I have been thinking whether I should register my idea or not? I need to see what I want from discussing my idea? Would I want the creation of the "trip to eternity" Institute and the "death card" to be with my permission? Do I want to get fame or wealth from registering my idea? Maybe sometime in the past I was interested in fame, but now I prefer to stay anonymous. If I could not think of writing this under a pen name, I would never have thought of writing it. And why did I decide to write this book? Why did I not start thinking about the investment part of it so that I could begin my institute sooner? Maybe my thought was more about creation of the idea and the expansion of it, and not about carrying out my idea.

I believe there are three types of people. First there are those who think and do, second those who cannot think but use the ideas of others, and third those who only think and do not do anything about it. I think I might belong to the third group. Constantly thinking of new ideas and necessary changes, but I would want to leave the actual execution to others. Now if they get lucky and someone comes their way and helps them, good, otherwise they would forget about doing anything. It may sound silly, but I have thought about putting an ad in the newspaper and renting my mental capacity and ideas. I would arrange it so that within the rental period for example one year, all of my ideas and thoughts would belong to someone else who can then invest upon them. But then I thought about writing and I realize that is something I am capable of doing easily. So that is how my book came about and I decided to leave the registration of my idea and the investment part of it to someone else.

"Part between part 12 and part 13"

Maybe it is time that I write this book in a different way, instead of just writing and typing up the words, to make an audiobook and to send that to a publisher. But I am not sure, is there a publisher who would accept an audiobook and not a written version? and I am not sure if I could record parts of my book and be able to correct them or not? I am not sure if I can publish an audiobook ? Turning the book into an audiobook and then giving a copy to be made for it to be turned into a pdf and then distributing that. They say lazy people become creative. They are right, but who said this? I do not know.

# Part 13

A few days ago when I was taking a break from writing, I started thinking about searching for investors. Who are they really? Would I go looking for them or do they have a nose for finding people with ideas? I would think that when there is the scent of money, they would come about, so maybe I would need to send out teasers to create interest. I would be able to tell them about my idea in brief. For example I can say: "If they invest in the creation of the travel to eternity Institute, for years they would be able to make money on their investments.

Why? Because in this institute the member's ages would be from 30 to 60 years old and the amount that they pay until the age of 80 would accumulate, and that is if they actually want to die at the age of 80, because some may change their minds and some may have already died for various reasons. This seems to be similar to how insurance works, so the investors would be able to make a good profit on their investment. Some may even join the institute at the age of 21 or above, which would yield better returns. Now that I think about it, I think maybe I should be the investor and make the profits myself! What would I want to consider, private investors or the government involvement if I choose to go that route? I think I prefer to go through a governmental institution, with the intent that this would lower the costs. But I am certain in the future, private institutions would be interested in these types of institutions. I have a feeling that the investors with their strong sense of making money would gather up.

## "Part between part 13 and part 14"

Many days have past and I have been writing without any worries about the type of the book or the style of my writing. But really, what type of a book would this become? Is this the kind of book that would just be a record of my daily ideas and if others want to pursue the ideas, they would be able to do so? With the creation of this institute a dream becomes a reality? Would this book become the kind that many would become interested in because they would want to find a way out of pain and suffering in their old age? Or would this book become like many others that will not find any readers? Would it become a best seller? Does anyone know what type of books become popular? Would having many readers, expand the sale of the book, or would advertising attract readers?

In my opinion in regard to the sale of books, a writer can write two types of books. One type would be books that would find many readers without anyone really knowing why? And the second type of books are those that spread quickly but the readership and sale of them is very slow. Books that no matter how much advertising is done, would not become too popular and sell well. So if a writer faces this type of difficulty, would have to forget the type of book that does not attract much attention and give up spending on advertising and other expenses, That writer would have to put that book aside and write a different book and come up with a different angle to present their idea. The writer would need to continue in order to find a type of a book that would spread quickly with many readers and good sales. That way with the fame and the proceeds from the book, that writer than can sell their previous works. The readers would then become interested in all their previously published books. But no one knows, neither the readers, nor the writers. Why?

Meanwhile if a writer after writing many pieces of work, becomes discouraged, or their mind becomes empty of ideas like a dry desert without any shrubs, and cannot write anymore or come up with any other ideas, would be able to take the previous works and write them differently. For example, turning a short story into a novel, or to write a different style of book going from serious to comedy or vice versa. because the technique of writing is really a way of playing with the words and the sentences. And skillfully with reading books, writing and publishing them, one becomes successful.

It is similar to when at the gathering, someone tells a joke and those around respond by laughing uncontrollably, but in another gathering if someone says the same joke, no one would even smile. Why? Is it the technique of telling the joke in the first speaker that the second person is unaware of? Does the first person have a certain skill that the second person lacks? Even though there is a technique and skill in telling a joke, sometimes it is not the speakers' skills that determines the successful outcome. Sometimes it has to do with who is telling the joke, their friends would laugh at anything they say whether it is funny or not. And there are those who when they speak, even if they say something funny, no one laughs at their jokes.

This is a similar problem with writers as well. Sometimes a good writer writes a very good book but cannot find many readers and cannot sell many books. In my opinion, for any book that is written, despite of the type of writing, the social situations, time, place, and advertising, would all affect it's success. And more than anything, it is the readers of those books depending on their situations and their ages, reading those books that determine their success and nothing else would affect success. I believe at the end everything must work, even the weather has something to do with the success of a book. I may need to have all the conditions to be right for my book to find readership, from time, place, societal conditions to even the weather. Or maybe not…. But I have a feeling that this book, no matter what the situation is, would encourage me to go on.

# Part 14

A few days ago I was talking to my father, and discussing my idea about the problems and issues with the old age, the idea of "the death card" and to having a choice that after the age of 80 legally being able to end our lives. My brother, who in hearing our conversations saw our father's interest in the subject said, maybe I would want to take care of dad to the age of 100 and it would not be important to me whether or not he has Alzheimer's or if he is incapacitated in any manner physically or mentally.

My father said kindly, you may want to be caring for me for a long time, but have you thought about what pains and sufferings I would endure? Do you know that when parents become old and incapable, how painful it is for them to see their children caring for them, and not just for a day or two, a week or two, but for months and years?

My brother became thoughtful, looking from my dad to me back-and-forth and said, but dad you may become old and even at the age of 90 enjoy being completely healthy. Would you want to die then?

In answer I told him, the person who is registered with the "trip to eternity" Institute and receives the "death card", only has the peace of mind that when they want, at any old age, to be able to choose to die. This does not mean that they cannot continue living and no laws would force them to die. This is just a choice, a legal death that anyone can choose for themselves at that time. That is all.

My brother began to understand and became pensive. I continued, it is similar to when someone writes a will, in regards to what happens to their possessions after their death. The "death card" is just like a will, where someone lets their children and relatives know when they reach an old age and if they suffer from Alzheimer's or become paralyzed, they would have the permission to allow them to die without any pain and suffering. It is only under the condition that if the old person becomes incapacitated, and is unable to speak, that it would take affect. My brother turned to my father and said, dad I really love you, but in reality it is not my choice and if you wish to die when you are older and incapable and do not want to continue living, it would be selfish for me to make you to live. Now that I think about it, I see that if you have chosen this for yourself, no one should prevent you to do as you wish especially if that is what you would want before you die. I suppose it is like when they want to carry out an execution, they ask a person for their last wish and they would respect that last wish. And maybe I would get the "death card" myself, even sooner than you. My father and I looked at each other and at him and smiled silently at each other.

"Part between part 14 and part 15"

I have been thinking that maybe I should write down my idea on a large piece of paper and carry it along with me wherever I go. Then anyone I speak to who would find this idea interesting and agree with, to sign the paper. But no that is an old way of doing things, maybe I should create a website, where others can consider the idea and vote.

Maybe if millions of people agree with this idea, then we can attract the government's attention and in a legal way create the "trip to eternity" Institute. Then for those who agree with me and myself, we can get "the death card".

# Part 15

PART 15

I would like to talk about some of the resources for this book, although it is customary that they are discussed at the end of the book, I think in regards to this book it does not make any difference. But in this case, it is more like a conversation and a bit of a friendly criticism.

One of my biggest difficulties is that I read several books at the same time and sometimes my mind is occupied with the writings from these books. It is not the details that occupy my mind, but it is the fact that I read sometimes four, eight, 16 or even 20 books at the same time, with apologies to those writers. Sometimes I wonder of the influence from those readings in my own writings. It doesn't matter to me where the writers are from, male or female, old, young or even a child, and what country and what religion they belong to. And so I do not know who or how to reference the book or the writer.

This may be a criticism of some writers who write books mostly by using the quotes from other books and writers. I am not sure are they trying to show their depth of knowledge by naming other books and writers or is it that do they lack any original thoughts, which would then remove the requirement of using other writer's works. It may be that if I were to look at it kindly, they are writers who have very good memories and they like to share the work of the other writers and it is not to be showing off!

So in this regard, it is my difficulty that I cannot reference the works of any other writers in writing my book. So I admit that in writing this book, I am using the writings of other writers along with references from movies and others resources indirectly. Can I pretend that this book is written solely from my own ideas and thoughts? Can any writer or inventor really claim that? Me? Who am I? How do you my ideas and thoughts form? Is it not that since childhood my mind has grown from observing others and what has gone on around me? From my parents, to my sister and brother, relatives, friends, enemies, the environment where I have lived, the weather, animals and plants, rivers and trees, all sources of energy visible or invisible, books and movies, and thousands of other things have gone hand-in-hand in order to make "me". These are the resources that have formed my thoughts and ideas, my likes and dislikes and have prepared me for writing this book. Maybe that is why I would like to write this book under a pen name of "a human". Because this book is being written by a human for other human beings, a human being, whose ideas have been formed by the thoughts and ideas of the others.

The good news is that in this case, no one would need to remember the name of the writer, especially the students whom the teachers constantly pressure to remember the names of the books, writers, the dates and places of birth,….. this was one of the issues I hated when I was at school, instead of concentrating on what the book was about when reading them, I had to memorize the names, dates of birth and death and other trivial details about their writers. So when others would ask me what the book was about, I would be stuck looking at them without having any idea about what I had read. I have no problem reading about the lives of the other writers and sometimes in order to get to know the origins of their psychology, I liked knowing the details of their lives, but after having paid enough attention to reading their works first. But I do not think a writer who does not reveal their name, would have any problem with that!

Is the existence or non-existence of a human being in the world full of people important? Are the thoughts of one human being amongst the thoughts of so many others important? Let us think about it…, would one human being on planet the earth, one human being in this world, one human being in between billions and billions of other humans matter? I feel so small and so insignificant.

No, Let us think about it differently. Let us think that the whole world is a "super human", and then imagine that every human being is a cell in the body of this "super human"… well, now it is better. Now if a cell does not do it's job well, what will happen? So every one human being is important. But in this view, is it important if it is a young and healthy human being or an old and incapable human being, who maybe paralyzed or be suffering from Alzheimer's and cannot continue living without the help of the others? I do not know where I have started from and where I am

going? This is how my mind likes to work, maybe it is right, maybe not…
My mind is like a small bird jumping from one branch to another branch,
but I think it is time that I stop my mind, do not continue in this path and
to force it to sit on one branch calmly. My poor small bird of a mind…

## "Part between part 15 and part 16"

A few days ago I was thinking about what type of life insurance I should get that would be better and more complete. I found an insurance that in addition to being a life insurance, included disability and coverage for the funeral expenses, and after 10 years it would pay interest. Of course most of my attention went to the disability part, which seemed to me comical. The way it was written was that if someone could not perform two of the four types of tasks, they would not be able to collect on this insurance. The four tasks included, if someone could not eat by themselves, use the bathroom, shower or walk by themselves.

I thought to myself, this is really silly, because if someone is not able to perform any of these tasks, they would be entitled to the long term disability insurance, if they have it, or is it not better for them to die. At least that is what I would choose. Of course someone would say, many choose to continue living even if they could not do any of these tasks, but thousands of like-minded people would agree with me. Of course I do not know really, which thousand people…!

I believe those who continue living in that manner, are doing so not of their own will, but are being made to do so by either their relatives or the law, and perhaps because they had not been able to arrange to end their pain and suffering in advance. I do not really know where we are going? Is it because we need to create jobs and there are those who want to make money, an arrangement by a system? In testing for new medications, do we need laboratory mice? Why can't we not use the old people who are at their deathbed and would not complain? Is there really no one else like me, who would want to have the "death card" for when it is necessary to die legally and without the pains and sufferings? Would it be a problem if I paid monthly dues to become a member of the "trip to eternity" institute so that when I am old and mentally or physically incapable, to end my life legally? Is it right that I, at an old age, while in pain and suffering constantly, to pay huge sums of money for medications, treatments, visits to the doctors, hospital stays and rest homes?

Is there not a problem with taking nature in our own hands and to lengthen the lives of the very old, who are incapable to live on their own, with the use of the medical technology? Would it be a problem to take nature in our own hands and with the injection of a strong calmative medication to end our pain and suffering at an old age with prior set up and request? Why is it legal to delay the death of the elderly, who are incapable of living on their own with the use of the medications, but it would not be illegal to speed up their death in a peaceful and calm manner with a simple injection voluntarily requested in advance?

If us humans choose to selfishly take nature in our own hands and lengthen the lives of the elderly, and to slow down their eventual death, then we should await the time when nature takes matters in hand and end the lives of the elderly in large numbers. Why? Because nature commands balance so the least we could do is to help the balance in nature by listening to the wishes of the elderly, to the wishes of the elderly who wish to slow down their death, while at the same time listening to those elderly people who would want to end their lives in a respectful and legal way and to help them quicken their death.

# Part 16

And now a trip to the future to see how everything would be since the establishment of the "trip to eternity" institute and as many people have their the "death cards". Many years has passed, we have aged and now that we want access to their services, what type of a building would we enter into? Maybe in the future others would have better ideas for the design of these buildings, but for now in my opinion we would need a building that would have three floors for the different types of people.

For sample I think we would need a lobby where people would enter. Maybe it is best we have the first floor for the people who are over 80 years old, those who are old and alone and do not want to continue living anymore. On this floor we would have beautifully designed rooms, such as in a five star hotel, for these people to spend their last few days and for their visitors and relatives to be able to come and say goodbye.

The second floor would be for those who are suffering from Alzheimer's or other mental ailments and/or are paralyzed, but would not need the help of doctors and nurses. On this floor, same as in the previous floor, we would have beautifully designed rooms that they would enter. Although many would not stay in these room for long, but maybe they would like to have their relatives who may have the same ideas and not want to continue living for too much longer to stay there.

The third floor would be for those who are 80 years old or older and for whatever ailment they may be suffering from, need to have the help of the doctors and nurses in their last few days. These people would have beautiful rooms as well so that if they still have some of their senses, they would enjoy their last few days and would feel safe and happy while they say goodbyes to their relatives.

But the basement would belong solely to those who are trained to work in this institution. They can only enter this space using biometrics, and from there they would have access to all the three floors so that they can carry out the dead and move them to the building behind the main building. Why have a building in the back? This would be a building that would be adjacent to the main building, but would only have access from the basement for transferring the bodies that would then be carried out for the funeral arrangements. These two buildings should have their separate entrances from two different streets, so that those who enter the first building would not encounter any of their outgoing bodies. I don't think it would be right for the people who enter the first building happily to be encountering the relatives of the dead who maybe sad or crying. And for those who are alone and do not have any friends and family, they can make all the arrangements so that after they enter the first building, the process of their funeral would be carried out step-by-step as they planned.

Now I want to see myself entering this building, I imagine myself old, more than 80 years old and alone, not having married and without any children, or if I have married and my spouse has passed away. whether I have children or not, they maybe living in various parts of the world. Since I no longer wish to continue my life, I would want to be welcomed by well mannered and kind individuals who would accompany me to my room. I would enter a beautiful room with a big window facing a beautiful garden. I would maybe call a friend or two to say goodbye or maybe not! I may want to listen to some pleasant music or maybe not! I may want to eat a delicious meal, or maybe not! After I have had my dinner, a few hours later, someone would inject me with a strong calmative medication, turn the TV on for me so that I can spend my last few moments watching some beautiful nature scenery and birds and slowly close my eyes and go to eternal sleep forever.

In the morning the doctor would arrive and would issue my death certificate and those who would be responsible for moving me to the basement, would arrive and remove my body and take it to the adjacent building, where my funeral procedure will be carried out as I had wished. I can not believe that such a day would come that my wish would be granted. Is it not our right to die when we want to, rather than the birth and death as it is now, where we have no control over? I am happy if I can see the day that I can choose to die when I want to, contrary to when I was born without having any choice.

## "Part between part 16 and part 17 (a)"

In the future if other creatures from other planets come to visit planet Earth, they would see the different institutions that have been set up so intelligently for those who would want to decide to end their lives for themselves. It would be interesting for them to see that human beings have decided to end their own lives when they are old and incapable or to continue their lives if they want to. Then in the cemeteries we would have new type of headstones that would have the birthdate, which was accidental, and the date of death, which would have been arranged. Of course there would be those who would die from accidental deaths, but such as it is now it would be a common incidence. It would not be any different than now and that would not be what happens to everyone.

## "Part between part 16 and part 17 (b)"

Sometimes I think to myself, should loneliness not be considered a type of illness? Is loneliness not a mental illness? If we choose to stay alone, are we then suffering from a mental illness or what if others leave us to be all alone?

There are times when we reach an old age, and would want to have connections to other people, but others would not for whatever reason stay connected and leave someone alone. Sometimes this loneliness goes on for a long time and would become a source of an illness. The lonely person would then lose their interest in living, even if they seem healthy and capable physically and mentally. Would the society, people, government and the law allow this old and lonely person to calmly and comfortably end their own life?

# Part 17

A while ago, I was talking to a friend who is familiar with my thoughts and ideas. She asked, have you thought about the bad things that may happen after you have shared your thoughts and ideas? After thinking for a while I answered, as you and I and everyone else know, when a new thought or idea has been presented, often things will happen that are beyond our control. When something happens, sometimes it is harmful to humans and sometimes it is to their benefit. It all depends on how a new idea is used. For example when knives were made, many used them in a many beneficial ways. When someone uses a knife to kill another, it does not take away from the benefit of the knife. Or with the invention of alcohol to serve humanity, some people drink a lot, drive under the influence and cause the death of themselves or others. This does not take away from the benefits of alcohol. Similarly when a man like Hitler comes up with the idea of bringing the world and many nations together with no borders, but goes about it in a way that causes the death of millions, his wrong actions do not detract from the correct and useful idea of universalization of all human beings.

With my ideas, when many elderly people who are incapable and alone and wish to die legally without pain and suffering, and someone come along and finds a way to benefit himself monetarily and force some older people to die sooner, is that not because of his ugly nature? Because there are those who find a way to benefit from any situation, it does not mean a useful idea should be questioned. My friend thought and said it looks like you have the answers to many of the issues and you have thoroughly thought about your idea! I said, it is true because I have been thinking about this for a long time and I wanted to make sure that I was not doing something wrong. Do you know why? Mostly because I have been thinking about this idea for myself and for when I become old and lonely and I believe that the laws should allow an older person to have a choice and to find a way to calmly die when they are ready. And of course I would not do something that would harm myself or bring about any harm to anyone else. I only want to be able to leave this world after living a happy and healthy life, that is all. Now in the future if others want to make the same choice, I would be happy.

## "Part between part 17 and part 18 (a)"

I am really happy to be writing this book under a pen name, one of the benefits of it is that when someone reads this book, they will read it for its own merits. Whether they like what is written or not, it would have nothing to do with who the writer is. I would prefer to stay anonymous, and until you have had that experience for yourself, you would not understand how it feels. I would recommend writing a book under a pseudonym to any writer so that they would experience the joy of just writing. it would be important to me to not be known in any gathering and to not have to travel all over to promote the book and to give talks. It has become customary for writers to go on a book tour and I dislike the idea and do not see the need for doing so.

We live in a world where everyone is constantly busy with their mobile phones and do not have any interest in listening and speaking to one another, and where everyone only uses their eyes to communicate rather than speaking to one another. Maybe in the future, many would lose their ability to speak and only a few would have preserved that ability. And similar to when we go to a concert and hear a singer, at that time people would gather to see someone who can speak because they have lost that ability themselves. They would look at the person who can speak with their jaws hanging open and would be confused on how that was happening! Let me see, have we already reached that age and we do not know it!? Is it not that when we go to a gathering where someone is speaking and all that they are saying is completely nonsense, do we not stand there and watch and listen without realizing it? So has this happened and we are not aware of it? Sometimes after going to a rally I think to myself, now I will listen carefully and when I do so, I realize most of what they are saying is completely nonsense. I realize that it is only the ambience of a big auditorium and the large number of the people gathered that had me under a spell to believe what the speaker was saying. I do not know what may have happened that I would have believed what was being said, and when I go back and listen to that speech a few times on my own, I realize that I did not believe what was being said. Do professional speakers use and play with our emotions?

## "Part between part 17 and part 18 (b)"

I believe our world has been in a standing still for a long time without many changes in regard to the birth and accidental death and we have no idea how to get away from the status quo. Maybe someone would come along and bring about some change and save us from repeating our actions over and over. Is it always that we have to wait for someone to come about and bring about change? What is the difference between you and I and those who come about and bring about change? Why can it not be you and I who can bring about change?

# Part 18

At few weeks ago enjoying a gathering with friends at a hall in a senior community, we entered after paying a small fee. Everyone brought their own food and drinks and enjoyed an indoor picnic and we drank, ate, listened to music and danced. There was a lot of positive energy all around. I slept really well that night, but in the morning, my heart was full of sadness thinking about the night before.

I tried to remember the night before, moment by moment, to see what had brought up the sadness. Suddenly I remembered that while sitting at a table enjoying ourselves, there was an old lady with dark glasses who asked if she could sit at one of the empty chairs at out table. She seemed full of sorrow and as we talked she told her tale of loneliness and of her various pains and aches, from her eyesight to her daily struggles.

You may think with my ideas I began talking to her about them, but no. I had two reasons for not speaking about my ideas. One was that I did not want to make her hopeful since it would take a long time for my plans to take shape and that would not benefit her. And two, because it cannot be only me, one person who advocates these ideas. It would take for many who believe in this idea to speak up and to help the elderly who are lonely and suffering. So I understood the reason for my sadness, realizing it was from putting myself in that woman's place and feeling her pain and sadness.

# PART 19

Some may have questions that if the elderly who are suffering from ailments, Alzheimer's and other mental and physical illnesses be able to die legally, how would that affect research, experimentations, scientists and doctors? How about the progress of the medical science, if that were the case?

In answer I would say and need to emphasize that by getting "the death card" and the death of the elderly and incapable people who choose to go this route, not everyone would then do so. As we know, human beings have different thoughts and desires and many do not even make simple plans for their future. Whether it be writing their will or planning for their funeral, so undoubtedly they would not get "the death card". These are the people that the scientist and doctors are continuously doing their research and experimentations on.

And I would like to discuss another point, and that is thinking that when I reach the age of 80 and even if I have obtained "the death card", can anyone force me to die at that age? Would the people around me force me to die? Would the law or the travel to eternity institute be able to force me to die? In answer I would say, absolutely not.

The person who becomes a member of the "trip to eternity" institute and receives "the death card", would only have the chance to choose the time of their death when they are ready. They can choose the time and to carry out their wishes to die if they choose to do so. It is similar to when someone after a lifetime of work, waiting to be retired can choose when to retire. Some choose to retire once they reach the retirement age, others choose to continue working. This is a choice for all human beings. That is all.

"Part between part 19 and 20 (a)"

So far I have presented my ideas and I have chosen to write them in the form of a book. That is what I am capable of doing for now, after the publication of my book, I would need to be patient and see what happens. I am a patient person and believe that when something is going to happen, it only takes for one person to take the first step and after that it is like the spark that begins a fire. This may be the spark that may begin a flame and then a fire in the jungle.

## "Part between part 19 and 20 (b)"

In the future I may choose to write a second, third or more volumes about my ideas. As long as my ideas flow I would write, even though I know in this day and age not many like to read books. These days fewer and fewer people have the patience to read books, and fewer and fewer people write letters, emails and telephone messages have become shorter and shorter. It seems like after many years of progress in writing, we are returning to the stone ages and the use of pictorial communications. More and more people only use emoji's to communicate, so maybe we would reach a day when if someone's grandfather passes away, they would only get pictures of the old man and his tombstone. They may then respond by sending a crying emoji to show their sorrow. Maybe they send several emoji's to communicate the depth of their despair. Knowing all this, I would still continue to write my books for those who still enjoy reading.

# Part 20

A few days ago a friend of mine was describing how her dog had fallen down the steps and had injured her back severely and of her plans to call an institution to come and put the dog down by injection of a calm active medication.

With a surprise I asked her does such an institute exist? She said of course, don't you know? With a smile I said no, I did not know!

As I was answering her, there was a joyfulness forming in my mind as I was thinking now that open minded people are accepting to put down their animals when they experience pain and suffering, then there is not a long before we can provide the same service for the old, incapable and lonely people.

Then I wondered, why had this not come to my mind before? So many things can be more comfortable and less expensive, and especially because for myself and those who think like me, I would not want us to pay high fees that would only fill the pockets of the institutions. So it is enough for a young person to join the "trip to eternity" institute, receive the "death card" and pay a small monthly fee, then when the time comes and we are old and incapable and need the services of this institute to be able to end our lives without any pain and suffering. My friend who saw me smiling asked, why what has happened to my dog making you smile?

Coming out of my daze I said, I am really sorry about your dog and for your loss, this is better than for your dog to suffer. I told her that I was thinking about something else when I smiled and that my mind was elsewhere. I told her about what I was thinking about, she smiled too and became pensive.

I told her I was happy that I had taken the first step by writing this book, presenting my idea and step-by-step going forward and that it seemed like there will be a path opening up for me, like always.

## "Part between part 20 and part 21"

I was editing my book when I noticed that inadvertently I had moved around some of the chapters and the in between chapters. For example, I had moved a chapter from the beginning to the end and had moved another chapter from the middle to the end and even some of the in between segments had been moved around and sometimes I needed to add or omit a segment and save it for book two. It occurred to me that what I was doing was similar to when someone is rearranging paintings in a gallery in order to make them flow and be seen better. Would moving paintings around in a gallery affect how the paintings are seen?

Would what I am doing influence how my readers read my book? Is it important that when entering a gallery, we start from one painting and move along one by one until we reach the end of the exhibit? Would we then be following the story that a painter is telling us? Would it not matter if we start from the end and move backwards as we view the paintings or if we start from the middle of the exhibit and move around without following any order? So if they would ask us to set up this exhibit, how would we organize the paintings? Maybe I would want to read my book in a certain order and another time I would want to read it a different way, and maybe the readers would want to move around as they read.

Has a writer ever written a best seller book and then changed it around to see what would happen if the order of the chapters were different? Would that make the book unpopular and unsuccessful or more successful and more popular? That is what happened in this book, so maybe if I go about editing a second or third time, the same thing may happen. Would it be possible for someone to not rearrange the paintings in a gallery as they set up the exhibit? It seems this book wants me to be writing it in this way, sometimes it is the writing that determines the flow for the writer, even if that seems unusual. In any event, as I have respect for my writing, I determine how the chapters and the in between segments should flow, but not a one hundred percent. Just as when events happen to us humans and we believe that we have control over our own lives, whereas we know we are following a certain faith even if not exactly one hundred percent.

# Part 21

I have a wish that I believe is the wish of many, I want there to be an institution where I could join and receive a card that would entitle me to be able to end my life legally when I am old, incapable and alone.

I have turned that wish into this book and I am releasing it into the ocean of the universe to do its job. My book would be like the famous corked bottle that someone has released into the ocean with my wish written on a piece of paper inside the bottle. This bottle will float around until someone finds it and recovers my plea for help. After writing this book, I would need to wait and see what happens. Would someone come to help me or would I be floating around like thousands in the ocean of hopelessness until my death?

I know when the time comes that one thing would lead to another so that my idea would reach the point where it can become a legal possibility. It seems like I am floating on the waves of the sea and those waves are leading me to shore. But if people need more time to understand and accept my idea, then there is nothing I can do and my push for it would not help. It may take many years or it may happen quickly so that happily we could have a choice at the time of our need and be able to die like a human being, and not like the critters that do not know when and where they would die. Like an out of control wheel birth and death, birth and death again in the endless cycle of …birth and death.

Would it not be possible for us to have a plan at the time of our birth, and to never have a plan to be able to have a choice for our death at the time when we are old? Many years has passed since we were a tiny being in this world? Now that we have grown up and have evolved, can we not have a choice about our own death at the time when we get old? Would there be a day when my wish could come true and for me to know that when I am old and when I want to, I can choose to legally die?

"The end"